HOPE DENNIS

Reverse Diabetes

Practical Strategies, Diet Changes, and Lifestyle Changes to Beat Diabetes

Contents

1

Introduction

A New Beginning: Reversing Type 2 Diabetes

For many diagnosed with type 2 diabetes, the condition can feel overwhelming and depressing. This book is going to show you that reversing your diabetes is not only possible, but it's also within your reach.

My name is Hope Dennis, and I was diagnosed with type 2 diabetes 12 years ago. I spent years researching and working with my doctor to help manage and reverse my diabetes. I wrote this book because everyone deserves to live a healthy, vibrant life, free from the constraints and complications of diabetes. Over the years, I've seen countless individuals transform their lives through practical strategies and lifestyle changes. The methods shared here are based on scientific research, real-life success stories, and my personal experiences with diabetes, just like you.

Why This Book Matters

You might be wondering, "Can I really reverse my diabetes?" The answer is yes. While diabetes is a serious condition, it's also one that can be managed and even reversed with the right approach. This book will provide you with a clear, step-by-step plan to help you achieve this goal. We'll cover everything from dietary changes and physical activity to medications, supplements, and self-care practices. Each chapter is designed to give you practical and actionable advice you can use immediately.

Type 2 diabetes doesn't have to control your life. With the information and strategies in this book, you can take control of your health and start living the life you've always wanted. This isn't about a quick fix or a fad diet. It's about making sustainable changes that will improve your health and well-being for the long term.

What You'll Learn

In the following chapters, we'll dive deep into understanding what type 2 diabetes is and how it develops. This foundational knowledge is crucial because it helps you understand why certain changes are necessary and how they will impact your health. You'll learn about the risk factors and causes of diabetes, the symptoms to watch for, and the potential complications if the condition is not managed properly.

Next, we'll explore the dietary changes that can help reverse diabetes. You'll discover which foods to avoid and which ones to embrace, how to plan your meals and the role of portion control. We'll also discuss the importance of physical activity and how incorporating regular exercise into your routine can dramatically improve your health.

In addition to diet and exercise, we'll look at medications and supplements that can support your journey to better health. While lifestyle changes are often the most effective way to manage diabetes, certain medications and supplements can provide additional support. We'll cover the options available and how to use them safely and effectively.

Monitoring your diabetes and practicing self-care are also crucial components of reversing the condition. You'll learn how to track your blood sugar levels, recognize warning signs, and make adjustments as needed. We'll provide tips on stress management, sleep hygiene, and other self-care practices that can help you stay on track.

Finally, we'll share tips and success stories from individuals who have successfully reversed their diabetes. These inspiring stories provide valuable insights and practical advice for your journey.

The Benefits of Reversing Diabetes

Reversing diabetes can have a profound impact on your life. Beyond the obvious health benefits, you'll likely experience increased energy levels, improved mood, and a greater sense of well-being. You'll reduce your risk of complications such as heart disease, kidney damage, and vision problems. And perhaps most importantly, you'll regain control over your health and your future.

Imagine enjoying your favorite activities without worrying about your blood sugar levels. Picture yourself feeling more confident, vibrant, and in tune with your body. Reversing diabetes has many benefits, and they are within your reach.

A Journey Worth Taking

Embarking on the journey to reverse diabetes is not always easy, but it is undoubtedly worth it. This book is your guide, providing you with the tools, knowledge, and support you need to succeed. Each chapter is designed to build on the previous one, creating a comprehensive roadmap to better health.

You don't have to navigate this journey alone. Throughout this book, you'll find practical advice, encouragement, and real-life examples to help you stay motivated and on track. Remember, the goal is not just to reverse diabetes but to create a healthier, more fulfilling life.

Transition to the Next Chapter

Now that we've set the stage, it's time to dive deeper. In the next chapter, we'll explore the fundamentals of type 2 diabetes, including how it develops and the factors that contribute to its onset. This understanding will provide a solid foundation for the practical strategies and lifestyle changes we'll discuss in later chapters.

Turn the page, and let's embark on this journey to better health together. Your new beginning starts now.

2

Chapter 1

Chapter 1: Understanding Type 2 Diabetes and How It Develops
Type 2 diabetes is a complex condition that affects millions of people worldwide. Understanding how it develops, recognizing its risk factors, symptoms, complications, and knowing how it is diagnosed are crucial steps toward managing and reversing it. In this chapter, we will explore these aspects in detail.

The Risk Factors and Causes of Type 2 Diabetes

Type 2 diabetes develops when the body becomes insulin resistant or the pancreas cannot produce enough insulin. Several factors contribute to the development of this condition, including:

1. **Genetic Factors**: A family history of diabetes increases the risk. If a parent or sibling has type 2 diabetes, the chances of developing the condition are higher.
2. **Lifestyle Factors**: Poor diet, lack of physical activity, and obesity are significant contributors. Diets high in refined sugars, fats, and processed foods can lead to weight gain and insulin resistance.
3. **Age**: The risk of type 2 diabetes increases, particularly after age 45. However, it is also diagnosed in younger populations, including

children, adolescents, and young adults.

4. **Ethnicity**: Certain ethnic groups, such as African Americans, Hispanics, Native Americans, and Asian Americans, are at higher risk.

5. **Medical Conditions**: Conditions like hypertension, abnormal cholesterol levels, and polycystic ovary syndrome (PCOS) can increase the risk.

6. **Other Factors**: Smoking, stress, and sleep disturbances are also linked to higher diabetes risk.

Understanding these risk factors helps recognize the changes needed to reduce the risk or manage the condition effectively.

The Symptoms of Type 2 Diabetes

Recognizing the symptoms of type 2 diabetes is crucial for early diagnosis and management. Common symptoms include:

1. **Frequent Urination**: Excess glucose in the bloodstream forces the kidneys to work harder to filter and absorb it, leading to frequent urination.

2. **Increased Thirst**: Frequent urination causes dehydration, which triggers intense thirst.

3. **Increased Hunger**: Despite eating, people with diabetes often feel hungry because their muscles and organs lack energy.

4. **Fatigue**: Insufficient sugar from the bloodstream into cells can lead to fatigue.

5. **Blurred Vision**: High blood sugar levels can pull fluid from the eyes' lenses, affecting vision.

6. **Slow-Healing Sores**: High blood sugar can affect blood flow and cause nerve damage, making it harder for the body to heal wounds.

7. **Frequent Infections**: Diabetes weakens the immune system, making infections more common.

The Risk Factors and Causes of Type 2 Diabetes

Type 2 diabetes develops due to genetic, environmental, and lifestyle factors. Understanding these risk factors and causes is crucial for managing and potentially reversing the condition. Here, we break down the primary contributors to the development of type 2 diabetes.

Genetic Factors

A family history of type 2 diabetes significantly increases your risk. If one or both of your parents or siblings have diabetes, your chances of developing the condition are higher. Genetic predisposition plays a role in how your body processes insulin and glucose.

Lifestyle Factors

Diet: Poor dietary choices are a leading cause of type 2 diabetes. Diets high in refined sugars, unhealthy fats, and processed foods contribute to weight gain and insulin resistance. Consuming large amounts of sugary drinks, fast food, and snacks with little nutritional value can lead to the development of diabetes.

Physical Inactivity: A sedentary lifestyle is another significant risk factor. Regular physical activity helps maintain a healthy weight, improves insulin sensitivity, and lowers blood sugar levels. Lack of exercise can contribute to weight gain and increase the risk of insulin resistance.

Obesity: Being overweight or obese is one of the most significant risk factors for type 2 diabetes. Excess fat, particularly abdominal fat, affects how your body uses insulin and processes glucose. Fat cells can release inflammatory chemicals that reduce the effectiveness of insulin.

Age

The risk of developing type 2 diabetes increases with age, particularly after 45. As you age, your body's efficiency in processing glucose can decline. However, the condition is becoming increasingly common in younger populations, including children and adolescents, mainly due to rising obesity rates and sedentary lifestyles.

Ethnicity

Certain ethnic groups are at a higher risk of developing type 2 diabetes. These groups include African Americans, Hispanics, Native Americans, and Asian Americans. Genetic predisposition and lifestyle factors in these communities contribute to the increased risk.

Medical Conditions

Prediabetes: Prediabetes is a condition where blood sugar levels are higher than normal but not yet high enough to be classified as diabetes. Without intervention, prediabetes often progresses to type 2 diabetes.

Polycystic Ovary Syndrome (PCOS): Women with PCOS, a condition characterized by hormonal imbalance and metabolism problems, have an increased risk of developing type 2 diabetes.

Hypertension: High blood pressure is commonly associated with type 2 diabetes. Both conditions share risk factors such as obesity and physical inactivity.

Cholesterol Levels: Abnormal cholesterol levels, deficient levels of high-density lipoprotein (HDL) cholesterol, and high levels of triglycerides can increase the risk of type 2 diabetes.

Other Factors

Smoking: Smokers are at a higher risk of developing type 2 diabetes than non-smokers. Smoking can increase inflammation, interfere with insulin effectiveness, and contribute to abdominal fat accumulation.

Stress: Chronic stress can lead to unhealthy behaviors such as overeating, lack of exercise, and poor sleep, all of which contribute to the risk of developing type 2 diabetes. Stress hormones can also interfere with insulin function.

Sleep Patterns: Poor sleep quality and irregular sleep patterns are linked to an increased risk of type 2 diabetes. Lack of sleep can affect insulin sensitivity and blood sugar levels.

Understanding these risk factors and causes can help you make informed decisions about your health. By addressing and modifying the factors within your control, such as diet, physical activity, and lifestyle habits, you can significantly reduce your risk of developing type 2 diabetes or manage the condition more effectively if you already have it.

Weight Loss: Some people lose weight despite eating more as their bodies turn to muscle and fat for energy.

Early detection of these symptoms can lead to prompt treatment and better management of the condition.

The Complications of Type 2 Diabetes

If left unmanaged, type 2 diabetes can lead to serious complications, including:

1. **Cardiovascular Disease**: Increased heart disease, stroke, and high blood pressure risk.
2. **Nerve Damage (Neuropathy)**: High blood sugar can injure the walls of the tiny blood vessels (capillaries) that nourish your nerves, particularly in the legs.
3. **Kidney Damage (Nephropathy)**: Diabetes can damage the delicate filtering system in the kidneys.
4. **Eye Damage (Retinopathy)**: Diabetes can damage the retina's blood vessels, potentially leading to blindness.
5. **Foot Damage**: Poor blood flow to the feet increases the risk of complications such as infections and poorly healing sores.
6. **Skin Conditions**: Diabetes may leave you more susceptible to skin problems, including bacterial and fungal infections.
7. **Hearing Impairment**: Hearing problems are more common in people with diabetes.
8. **Alzheimer's Disease**: Type 2 diabetes may increase the risk of dementia, including Alzheimer's disease.

Awareness of these complications emphasizes the importance of managing blood sugar levels effectively to prevent long-term damage.

The Diagnosis of Type 2 Diabetes

Diagnosis of type 2 diabetes involves several tests:

1. **Glycated Hemoglobin (A1C) Test**: This test measures the average blood sugar level for the past two to three months. An A1C level of 6.5% or higher on two separate tests indicates diabetes.
2. **Random Blood Sugar Test**: A blood sample taken at a random time. A random blood sugar level of 200 mg/dL or higher suggests diabetes.
3. **Fasting Blood Sugar Test**: A blood sample taken after an overnight fast. A fasting blood sugar level of less than 100 mg/dL is normal, 100 to 125 mg/dL indicates prediabetes, and 126 mg/dL or higher on two separate tests indicates diabetes.
4. **Oral Glucose Tolerance Test**: This test involves fasting overnight, then drinking a sugary liquid and measuring blood sugar levels periodically for the next two hours. A blood sugar level of 200 mg/dL or higher after two hours indicates diabetes.

Early and accurate diagnosis is essential for effective management and reversal of type 2 diabetes.

Conclusion

Understanding type 2 diabetes and how it develops is the first step towards managing and potentially reversing it. By recognizing the risk factors, symptoms, complications, and diagnostic methods, you are better equipped to take proactive steps toward better health. The next chapter will delve into the dietary changes necessary to reverse diabetes, providing practical guidelines and tips to transform your eating habits. Let's move forward on this journey to improved health together.

The Risk Factors and Causes of Type 2 Diabetes

Type 2 diabetes develops due to genetic, environmental, and lifestyle factors. Understanding these risk factors and causes is crucial for managing and potentially reversing the condition. Here, we break down the primary contributors to the development of type 2 diabetes.

Genetic Factors

Family History: A family history of type 2 diabetes significantly increases your risk. If one or both of your parents or siblings have diabetes, your chances of developing the condition are higher. Genetic predisposition plays a role in how your body processes insulin and glucose. While you cannot change your genetic makeup, knowing your family history can help you take proactive steps to reduce other modifiable risk factors.

Genetic Predispositions: Some individuals inherit genes that make them more susceptible to developing type 2 diabetes. These genes can affect how the body produces and uses insulin, leading to insulin resistance or decreased insulin production.

Lifestyle Factors

Diet: Poor dietary choices are a leading cause of type 2 diabetes. Diets high in refined sugars, unhealthy fats, and processed foods contribute to weight gain and insulin resistance. Consuming large amounts of sugary drinks, fast food, and snacks with little nutritional value can lead to the development of diabetes. Key dietary contributors include:

- **High Sugar Intake**: Frequent consumption of sugary beverages and snacks spikes blood sugar levels, leading to insulin overproduction and eventual insulin resistance.
- **High Fat Intake**: Diets rich in saturated and trans fats contribute to weight gain and impair insulin sensitivity.
- **Low Fiber Intake**: Fiber helps regulate blood sugar levels. Diets low in fruits, vegetables, whole grains, and legumes can lead to poor blood sugar control.

Physical Inactivity: A sedentary lifestyle is another significant risk factor. Regular physical activity helps maintain a healthy weight, improves insulin sensitivity, and lowers blood sugar levels. Lack of exercise can contribute to weight gain and increase the risk of insulin resistance. Physical activity helps muscles use glucose more effectively, reducing blood sugar levels.

Obesity: Being overweight or obese is one of the most significant risk factors for type 2 diabetes. Excess fat, particularly abdominal fat, affects how your body uses insulin and processes glucose. Fat cells can release inflammatory chemicals that reduce the effectiveness of insulin. Key points include:

- **Visceral Fat**: Fat around the abdominal organs (visceral fat) is harmful and associated with insulin resistance.
- **Body Mass Index (BMI)**: A higher BMI correlates with an increased risk of developing type 2 diabetes. However, even modest weight loss can significantly reduce this risk.

Age

The risk of developing type 2 diabetes increases with age, particularly after 45. As you age, your body's efficiency in processing glucose can decline. However, the condition is becoming increasingly common in younger populations, including children and adolescents, mainly due to rising obesity rates and sedentary lifestyles. Aging affects the body's ability to produce and use insulin effectively, making older adults more susceptible.

Ethnicity

Certain ethnic groups are at a higher risk of developing type 2 diabetes. These groups include African Americans, Hispanics, Native Americans, and Asian Americans. Genetic predisposition and lifestyle factors are prevalent in these communities, contributing to the increased risk. Social determinants of health, such as access to healthcare, socioeconomic status, and cultural dietary practices, also play a role.

Medical Conditions

Prediabetes: Prediabetes is a condition where blood sugar levels are higher than normal but not yet high enough to be classified as diabetes. Without intervention, prediabetes often progresses to type 2 diabetes. Lifestyle changes such as improved diet and increased physical activity can prevent the progression.

Polycystic Ovary Syndrome (PCOS): Women with PCOS, a condition characterized by hormonal imbalance and metabolism problems, have an increased risk of developing type 2 diabetes. PCOS is associated with insulin resistance, which can lead to higher blood sugar levels.

Hypertension: High blood pressure is commonly associated with type 2 diabetes. Both conditions share risk factors such as obesity and physical inactivity. Hypertension can damage blood vessels and contribute to insulin resistance.

Cholesterol Levels: Abnormal cholesterol levels, deficient levels of high-density lipoprotein (HDL) cholesterol, and high levels of triglyc-erides can increase the risk of type 2 diabetes. These lipid abnormalities can also lead to insulin resistance and cardiovascular disease.

Other Factors

Smoking: Smokers are at a higher risk of developing type 2 diabetes than non-smokers. Smoking can increase inflammation, interfere with insulin effectiveness, and contribute to abdominal fat accumulation. Nicotine can alter glucose metabolism and increase insulin resistance.

Stress: Chronic stress can lead to unhealthy behaviors such as overeat-ing, lack of exercise, and poor sleep, all of which contribute to the risk of developing type 2 diabetes. Stress hormones like cortisol can also interfere with insulin function and increase blood sugar levels.

Sleep Patterns: Poor sleep quality and irregular sleep patterns are linked to an increased risk of type 2 diabetes. Lack of sleep can affect insulin sensitivity and blood sugar levels. Sleep deprivation can disrupt the balance of hormones that regulate hunger and appetite, leading to overeating and weight gain.

Understanding these risk factors and causes can help you make informed decisions about your health. By addressing and modifying the factors within your control, such as diet, physical activity, and lifestyle habits, you can significantly reduce your risk of developing type 2 diabetes or manage the condition more effectively if you already have it. This comprehensive approach to understanding the disease's development sets the foundation for the practical strategies discussed in the following chapters.

The Symptoms of Type 2 Diabetes

Recognizing the symptoms of type 2 diabetes is critical for early diagnosis and effective management. Often, symptoms develop gradually, which can make them easy to overlook. Here are the key symptoms typically associated with type 2 diabetes:

Increased Thirst and Frequent Urination: High blood sugar levels cause the kidneys to work harder to filter and absorb excess glucose. When the kidneys can't keep up, the excess glucose is excreted into the urine, pulling fluids from your tissues. This process leads to dehydration, making you thirsty and causing you to drink and urinate more frequently.

Increased Hunger: Despite eating, you may feel constantly hungry. This is because the body's cells do not receive enough energy glucose due to insulin resistance. As a result, the body signals the need for more food, trying to obtain energy from new food intake.

Fatigue: High blood sugar levels can affect your body's ability to convert glucose into energy efficiently, leaving you feeling fatigued. This can be exacerbated by dehydration from frequent urination.

Blurred Vision: In the short term, high blood sugar levels can cause fluid to be pulled from the lenses of your eyes, affecting your ability to focus and blurring your vision. If blood sugar levels fluctuate often, these changes in fluid levels can lead to vision issues.

Slow-Healing Sores and Frequent Infections: High blood sugar levels impair the body's natural healing process and reduce the ability to fight infections. Cuts and sores heal slowly, and individuals may experience frequent infections, particularly in the skin or urinary tract.

Numbness or Tingling in Hands and Feet: Excess sugar in the bloodstream can cause nerve damage over time, leading to a condition known as neuropathy. Neuropathy can manifest as tingling, numbness, or pain in the extremities, especially in the hands and feet.

Darkened Skin in Certain Areas: Some people with type 2 diabetes develop patches of darkened skin, particularly in the neck and armpit areas. This condition, known as acanthosis nigricans, is a sign of insulin resistance.

Unexplained Weight Loss: In some cases, despite eating more to relieve hunger, weight loss may occur. When insulin cannot effectively transport glucose into the cells, the body begins to break down fat and muscle for energy, leading to weight loss.

Irritability and Other Mood Changes: Fluctuations in blood sugar levels can also affect your mood and mental state, leading to irritability and other changes that might not be easily explained by different factors in your life.

These symptoms can also be related to other conditions, so experiencing them does not necessarily mean you have diabetes. However, seeing a healthcare provider for evaluation is important if you notice one or more of these symptoms. Early detection can lead to better management of the condition and help prevent the development of serious complications associated with diabetes.

The Complications of Type 2 Diabetes

Type 2 diabetes can lead to a wide range of complications if not managed properly. These complications can affect nearly every organ in the body, resulting in significant health problems that can impact quality of life and overall health. Here is a straightforward breakdown of the major complications associated with type 2 diabetes:

Cardiovascular Disease: Diabetes dramatically increases the risk of various cardiovascular problems, including coronary artery disease with chest pain (angina), heart attack, stroke, and narrowing of arteries (atherosclerosis). Diabetes leads to changes in the blood vessels, such as stiffening or thickening, which can impede blood flow, increasing the risk of vascular disease.

Nerve Damage (Neuropathy): Excess glucose in the blood can injure the walls of tiny blood vessels (capillaries) that nourish your nerves, especially in the legs. This can cause tingling, numbness, burning, or pain that usually begins at the tips of the toes or fingers and gradually spreads upwards. You could lose all sense of feeling in the affected limbs if untreated.

Kidney Damage (Nephropathy): The kidneys contain millions of tiny blood vessel clusters that filter waste from your blood. Diabetes can damage this delicate filtering system, leading to severe kidney damage or even kidney failure, requiring dialysis or a kidney transplant.

Eye Damage (Retinopathy): Diabetes can damage the retina's blood vessels (diabetic retinopathy), potentially leading to blindness. Diabetes also increases the risk of other serious vision conditions, such as cataracts and glaucoma.

Foot Damage: Nerve damage in the feet or poor blood flow to the feet increases the risk of various foot complications. Left untreated, cuts and blisters can become serious infections, which may heal poorly. Severe damage might require toe, foot, or leg amputation.

Skin Conditions: Diabetes may leave you more susceptible to skin problems, including bacterial and fungal infections.

Hearing Impairment: Hearing problems are more common in people with diabetes, possibly due to nerve damage affecting the ears or poor circulation.

Alzheimer's Disease: Type 2 diabetes seems to increase the risk of Alzheimer's disease and other dementias. Poor blood sugar control is linked to quicker cognitive decline.

Depression: The rigors of managing chronic diabetes can contribute to the onset of depression, which can, in turn, make diabetes management more challenging.

Sleep Apnea: People with type 2 diabetes often have sleep apnea, which causes breathing to stop and start during sleep. This condition can worsen diabetes control and increase the risks of cardiovascular disease.

These complications highlight the importance of managing diabetes through lifestyle changes, medication, and monitoring. Effective management can help prevent or delay these complications and contribute to a healthier, longer life. If you have type 2 diabetes, regular follow-up with health care providers and adherence to treatment plans are crucial for preventing these serious complications.

The Diagnosis of Type 2 Diabetes

Diagnosing type 2 diabetes involves several tests that measure your blood sugar levels. These tests are crucial for detecting the condition early and starting effective management to prevent complications. Here is an overview of the key diagnostic tests used to confirm type 2 diabetes:

Glycated Hemoglobin (A1C) Test: This test measures your average blood glucose levels over the past 2 to 3 months. It checks the percentage of blood sugar attached to hemoglobin, the oxygen-carrying protein in red blood cells. An A1C level of 6.5% or higher on two separate occasions indicates diabetes. Levels between 5.7% and 6.4% suggest prediabetes.

Fasting Blood Sugar Test: This test measures your blood sugar after an overnight fast. A fasting blood sugar level of 126 milligrams per deciliter (mg/dL) or higher on two separate tests confirms diabetes. Levels from

100 to 125 mg/dL indicate prediabetes.

Oral Glucose Tolerance Test (OGTT): After fasting overnight, you drink a sugary liquid, and your blood sugar levels are tested periodically over the next two hours. A blood sugar level of 200 mg/dL or higher after two hours points to diabetes. Levels between 140 and 199 mg/dL indicate prediabetes.

Random Blood Sugar Test: This test measures your blood sugar at any time, regardless of when you last ate. A blood sugar level of 200 mg/dL or higher suggests diabetes, especially if accompanied by symptoms of the disease, such as frequent urination, increased thirst, and unexplained weight loss.

These diagnostic tests help healthcare providers determine not only if you have diabetes but also how well you're managing the disease if you've already been diagnosed. Early and accurate diagnosis is essential for managing diabetes effectively, reducing the risk of complications, and improving overall health outcomes. If you exhibit symptoms of diabetes or have risk factors for the disease, undergoing one or more of these tests is critical.

3

Chapter 2

Chapter 2: **Dietary Changes Needed to Reverse Diabetes**

Managing and potentially reversing type 2 diabetes can significantly depend on dietary habits. This chapter will delve into how dietary changes can help control blood sugar levels, improve overall health, and reverse diabetes symptoms over time. It will cover the role of diet in managing diabetes, the importance of choosing the right foods, which foods to avoid, and practical tips for portion control and meal planning.

Overview of the Roles of Dieting for Reversing Type 2 Diabetes

Diet plays a crucial role in managing type 2 diabetes. What you eat directly impacts your blood sugar levels, body weight, and heart health—all key factors in diabetes management. A proper diet helps stabilize blood sugar levels, reduces the risk of complications, and can even reverse diabetes progression. This section will explore how diet affects glucose metabolism and insulin sensitivity and how making the right dietary choices can be as powerful as medication.

The Importance of a Healthy Diet for Type 2 Diabetes

A healthy diet is essential not just for managing blood sugar but also for maintaining overall well-being. For individuals with type 2 diabetes, a healthy diet can help manage body weight, reduce inflammation, and lower the risk of heart disease. This section will detail the components of a diabetes-friendly diet, such as high fiber content, low glycemic index foods, and balanced macronutrients, and explain how these components work together to help manage diabetes.

The Foods to Avoid and Include in a Diabetes-Friendly Diet

Foods to Avoid:

- **High Sugar Foods:** Sodas, desserts, and candies can cause blood sugar spikes.
- **Refined Carbs:** White bread, pasta, and anything made with white flour have high glycemic indexes.
- **Trans Fats and High Saturated Fats:** Margarine, fried foods, and high-fat dairy products can worsen heart health.
- **Processed Meats:** These are often high in sodium and unhealthy fats.

Foods to Include:

- **Fiber-Rich Foods:** Vegetables, fruits, legumes, and whole grains help control blood sugar levels.
- **Lean Proteins:** Fish, chicken, and plant-based proteins support muscle health without impacting glucose levels.
- **Healthy Fats:** Nuts, seeds, avocados, and olive oil can help maintain blood sugar levels.
- **Low Glycemic Index Fruits:** Berries, apples, and pears offer sweetness without causing significant glucose spikes.

This section will provide a detailed list of foods to avoid and encourage and explain how certain foods affect blood sugar levels, body weight, and overall health.

Portion Control and Meal Planning

Mastering portion control and meal planning is crucial for keeping blood sugar levels stable throughout the day. This section will offer strategies for portion control, such as using smaller plates, reading food labels, and understanding serving sizes. It will also cover how to plan meals throughout the day to prevent spikes and drops in blood sugar levels, including the importance of consistent meal timing, incorporating a variety of nutrients in meals, and adjusting portions based on activity levels and metabolic needs.

Meal-planning tips include preparing meals ahead of time, making smart choices when dining out, and maintaining a balanced diet while still enjoying food. This section will provide practical advice, tools, and sample meal plans to help readers implement these strategies into their daily lives.

By the end of this chapter, readers will have a thorough understanding of the dietary changes necessary to manage and potentially reverse type 2 diabetes. They will be equipped with the knowledge to make informed decisions about what, when, and how much to eat to maintain stable blood sugar levels and support overall health.

Overview of the Roles of Dieting for Reversing Type 2 Diabetes

Diet plays a fundamental role in the management and potential reversal of type 2 diabetes. It is one of the most effective tools to influence blood sugar levels, insulin sensitivity, and overall metabolic health. Understanding the impact of diet on diabetes is crucial for anyone looking to mitigate their symptoms or reverse the course of their condition. This section explores how strategic dietary choices can profoundly affect diabetes.

Blood Sugar Regulation: The primary goal of dietary management in type 2 diabetes is to maintain stable blood sugar levels. Foods high in refined sugars and carbohydrates can cause rapid spikes in blood glucose, which can be harmful over time. By choosing foods with a low glycemic index, which release sugar into the bloodstream more slowly, you can help maintain more consistent blood sugar levels, reducing the risk of hyperglycemia and providing better overall glucose control.

Insulin Sensitivity Improvement: Diet also significantly affects insulin sensitivity. Consuming a diet high in saturated and trans fats can increase insulin resistance, where the body's cells do not respond adequately to insulin. In contrast, diets rich in omega-3 fatty acids, fiber, and healthy fats can enhance insulin sensitivity. Improved insulin sensitivity means that the body can more effectively use the insulin it produces, which is crucial for managing blood sugar levels.

Weight Management: For many individuals with type 2 diabetes, achieving and maintaining a healthy weight is vital. Excess body fat, especially around the waist, is linked to increased insulin resistance. A diet that promotes a healthy weight can help decrease body fat, reduce insulin resistance, and lower the risk of developing complications associated with diabetes.

Reducing Complications: A well-planned diet can also help prevent or manage the myriad complications associated with diabetes, such as heart disease, kidney damage, and nerve damage. Diets low in sodium and unhealthy fats but rich in antioxidants and phytochemicals from fruits and vegetables can protect the body's tissues from diabetes-related damage and reduce inflammation.

Holistic Health Improvement: Beyond directly impacting glucose metabolism and diabetes symptoms, diet enhances overall health. A nutritious diet supports cardiovascular health, improves energy levels, enhances mental well-being, and strengthens the immune system. These benefits are significant for individuals with chronic conditions like diabetes, as they can significantly influence the quality of life and overall longevity.

In summary, dieting intending to reverse type 2 diabetes is not just about restricting certain foods but about creating a balanced, nutritious eating plan that supports stable blood sugar levels, improves insulin sensitivity, promotes a healthy weight, reduces the risk of complications, and enhances overall health. The following sections will detail specific dietary strategies, including which foods to avoid and include and how to implement effective portion control and meal planning.

The Importance of a Healthy Diet for Type 2 Diabetes

A healthy diet is essential for managing type 2 diabetes effectively. It impacts not only blood sugar levels but also overall health and well-being. This subsection outlines the key reasons why maintaining a healthy diet is crucial for individuals with type 2 diabetes.

Stabilizes Blood Sugar Levels: A well-balanced diet helps stabilize blood sugar levels by providing a steady energy source throughout the day. Foods that are low in glycemic index and high in fiber slow down the absorption of sugar in the bloodstream, preventing spikes and crashes that can complicate diabetes management.

Improves Insulin Sensitivity: Eating the right mix of foods can improve insulin sensitivity, which means the body's cells can better use available insulin to absorb glucose from the bloodstream. Foods rich in healthy fats, like omega-3 fatty acids from fish and monounsaturated fats from nuts and avocados, and moderate exercise can enhance insulin sensitivity.

Reduces Body Fat: A healthy diet is pivotal in weight management, particularly in controlling type 2 diabetes. Excess body fat, especially around the abdomen, increases insulin resistance. Managing dietary intake helps reduce and control weight, thereby improving diabetes outcomes.

Lower Risk of Complications: Type 2 diabetes is associated with several health complications, including cardiovascular disease, kidney damage, and nerve damage. A diet low in saturated fats, trans fats, and cholesterol, but rich in fruits, vegetables, and whole grains can help reduce the risk of these complications by promoting better blood pressure and cholesterol levels.

Enhances Overall Well-being: A nutritious diet enhances overall physical health, boosts energy levels, and can improve mood and mental health. For individuals with type 2 diabetes, this can mean better daily management of their condition, less fatigue, and a reduced risk of depression.

Supports Long-term Health: Consistently following a healthy diet helps establish long-term habits crucial for managing diabetes. It can lead to sustained improvements in blood sugar control, reduced medication need, and a better quality of life.

In summary, the importance of a healthy diet in managing type 2 diabetes cannot be overstated. It is a foundational component of diabetes care that directly affects glucose control, weight management, prevention of complications, and overall health enhancement. Making informed dietary choices is not just about avoiding unhealthy foods but about integrating a balanced, nutritious approach to eating that supports long-term diabetes management and overall health.

The Foods to Avoid and Include in a Diabetes-Friendly Diet

Managing type 2 diabetes effectively requires careful attention to your diet. Knowing which foods to avoid and which to include can significantly influence your blood sugar levels and overall health. Here's a concise guide to help you make informed choices about your diet.

Foods to Avoid

High-Sugar Foods and Beverages: Avoid sugary drinks like sodas, fruit punches, and energy drinks, as well as sweets like candy, cakes, and ice cream. These foods cause rapid spikes in blood glucose levels.

Refined Carbohydrates: White bread, white rice, pastries, and other baked goods made from refined flour have a high glycemic index and can quickly elevate blood sugar levels.

Trans Fats: Artificial trans fats are harmful in margarine, peanut butter, spreads, and some packaged snacks. They contribute to heart disease, which people with diabetes are at higher risk for.

High-Fat Animal Products: Limit or avoid high-fat cuts of meat, such as ribs and bacon, and full-fat dairy products. These foods are rich in saturated fats, which can worsen insulin resistance.

Fried Foods: Deep-fried foods absorb a lot of fat during cooking, which can lead to weight gain and increased cholesterol levels.

Highly Processed Foods: These often contain unhealthy fats, sugars, and sodium. Always read labels to check for hidden sugars and fats in packaged foods.

Foods to Include

Fiber-Rich Foods: Incorporate plenty of fiber into your diet, as it helps slow down glucose absorption. Good sources include vegetables, fruits, legumes, and whole grains like quinoa and oats.

Lean Proteins: Include lean protein sources to help manage hunger without affecting blood sugar levels. Options include chicken, turkey, fish, eggs, and plant-based proteins like tofu and tempeh.

Healthy Fats: Foods rich in healthy fats can help improve blood cholesterol levels and maintain cell health. Include avocados, nuts, seeds, and olive oil in your diet.

Fresh Fruits: While fruit contains sugar, it also has fiber and numerous vitamins. Choose fresh fruits like berries, apples, and oranges over juices.

Non-Starchy Vegetables: These are low in carbohydrates and calories but high in vitamins and minerals. Include a variety of colors in your diet with vegetables like leafy greens, peppers, and broccoli.

Low-Fat Dairy or Plant-Based Alternatives: These can provide calcium and protein without the high-fat content. Choose low-fat milk, cheese, yogurt, or plant-based alternatives like almond or soy milk.

In summary, a diabetes-friendly diet should minimize the intake of high-glycemic, processed, and high-fat foods while emphasizing fiber-rich, whole, and nutrient-dense foods. This balanced approach helps manage blood sugar levels, promotes a healthy weight, and reduces the risk of diabetes-related complications.

Portion Control and Meal Planning

Diligent portion control and strategic meal planning greatly enhance the effective management of type 2 diabetes. These practices help regulate blood sugar levels, manage caloric intake, and promote overall health. Here's a detailed approach to mastering portion control and meal planning for optimal diabetes management.

Portion Control

Use Smaller Plates: Switching to smaller plates can trick your mind into thinking that you are eating more than you are, helping to reduce overall calorie intake without feeling deprived.

Read Nutrition Labels: Understanding nutrition labels is crucial. Pay attention to serving sizes and the number of servings per container. Use measuring cups or a digital scale to ensure you are eating exactly one serving, or adjust according to your dietary needs.

Divide Your Plate Methodically: Adopt the plate method for a balanced diet—half the plate filled with non-starchy vegetables (like spinach, carrots, and broccoli), one quarter with high-quality protein (such as grilled chicken or tofu), and the remaining quarter with complex carbohydrates (like brown rice or sweet potatoes).

Avoid Eating from the Package: Directly eating from a package can lead to overeating. Instead, portion out snacks or meals into a bowl or plate to avoid consuming more than intended.

Listen to Your Hunger Cues: Eat slowly and stop eating when full. It takes about 20 minutes for your brain to register fullness from the stomach, so give yourself time to feel satiated.

Meal Planning

Plan Your Meals Weekly: Sit down once a week to plan your meals. Planning your meals helps you maintain a balanced diet, manage portions, and avoid the temptation of unhealthy foods. It also makes grocery shopping more efficient and can reduce food waste.

Ensure Nutritional Balance: Each meal should be balanced to slow glucose absorption and control blood sugar levels. Include a mix of low glycemic index carbohydrates, fiber, lean proteins, and healthy fats in each meal.

Consistent Meal Timing: Eat your meals and snacks simultaneously daily to stabilize your blood sugar levels. Consistency is key in preventing spikes and crashes, especially if you are on medications or insulin.

Prepare Meals in Advance: Use your meal plan to prepare meals ahead of time. Batch cooking and portion-controlled containers can help you stick to your diet plan, especially during busy days.

Smart Snacking: Incorporate snacks into your meal plan to manage hunger and prevent overeating at mealtime. Choose snacks rich in fiber and protein, such as an apple with almond butter, a small portion of nuts, or raw vegetables with hummus.

Adjust Portions Based on Activity Levels: If you are more active on certain days, plan to include more carbohydrates to keep your energy levels up. Conversely, on less active days, reduce carbohydrate intake to prevent high blood sugar levels.

Regular Monitoring: Monitor your blood sugar responses to different meals. This can help you fine-tune your meal plan and portion sizes to better manage your diabetes.

By enhancing your portion control and meal planning skills, you can make significant strides in managing your type 2 diabetes effectively. These practices not only aid in maintaining stable blood sugar levels, support sustainable weight management, and contribute to overall health and well-being.

Chapter 3

Chapter 3: **Physical Activity and Exercise for Reversing Diabetes**
The role of physical activity in managing and reversing type 2 diabetes cannot be overstated. This chapter delves into how regular exercise can significantly improve blood sugar control, enhance insulin sensitivity, and improve overall health. Effective exercise strategies tailored specifically for individuals with type 2 diabetes are essential for harnessing these benefits.

The Benefits of Exercise for Reversal of Type 2 Diabetes

Improves Insulin Sensitivity: Regular physical activity helps your muscles use blood glucose for energy more efficiently, which improves insulin sensitivity. This means that your body will require less insulin to control blood sugar levels after periods of regular exercise.

Aids in Weight Management: Exercise is key to losing weight and maintaining a healthy weight, which is crucial for managing diabetes. Reducing body fat, especially around the abdomen, decreases the body's resistance to insulin.

Lowers Blood Sugar Levels: Physical activity helps to lower blood sugar levels during and after exercise. Regular exercise can help to stabilize your blood sugar levels over time.

Reduces Cardiovascular Risk: People with diabetes are at increased risk for cardiovascular diseases. Exercise improves heart health by lowering blood pressure, improving cholesterol levels, and strengthening the heart muscle.

Enhances Overall Well-Being: Exercise releases endorphins, natural mood lifters, which can help alleviate stress and depression, common challenges for those managing chronic conditions like diabetes.

Types of Exercises for Type 2 Diabetes

Aerobic Exercise: Walking, swimming, running, and cycling can significantly lower blood sugar levels. Aim for at least 150 minutes of moderate to vigorous aerobic activity weekly.

Resistance Training: Lifting weights or using resistance bands can improve strength, balance, and the ability to manage diabetes. Muscles are good metabolizers of glucose, and building muscle mass helps your body regulate blood sugar more efficiently.

Flexibility Exercises: Stretching and exercises like yoga and Pilates improve flexibility, range of motion, and blood flow. They also reduce stress, which can help control blood glucose levels.

Balance Training: Activities that improve balance, such as tai chi, can help prevent falls, which is particularly important as people with diabetes may have nerve damage in their feet.

Starting an Exercise Plan

Consult Your Doctor: Before starting any new exercise regimen, discuss it with your healthcare provider, especially if you have existing health concerns or complications associated with diabetes.

Start Slow: Begin with low-intensity activities and gradually increase intensity and duration to avoid hypoglycemia, especially if you are on insulin or other medications that increase insulin production.

Monitor Blood Sugar Levels: Check your blood sugar before, during, and after exercise to understand how you respond to different activities and to prevent dangerous blood sugar fluctuations.

Stay Hydrated: Staying hydrated helps modulate blood sugar levels and prevent dehydration, especially if your blood sugar levels are higher.

Pointers to Stay Motivated to Exercise Regularly

Set Realistic Goals: Create achievable goals that motivate you and celebrate milestones, no matter how small.

Find Activities You Enjoy: Exercise doesn't have to be a chore. Finding activities you love increases the likelihood that you'll stick with them.

Build a Support Network: Exercise with friends, join a class, or participate in a community with similar health goals to increase your motivation.

Track Your Progress: Use a journal or app to monitor your progress and improvements. Seeing actual progress can be a powerful motivator.

Incorporate Variety: Keep your routine interesting by trying new exercises or activities to avoid boredom and hitting a plateau in your progress.

By understanding the pivotal role of exercise in diabetes management, integrating it into your daily routine, and maintaining motivation, you can significantly enhance your ability to manage and potentially reverse type 2 diabetes. This chapter aims to provide the knowledge and tools needed to make physical activity a cornerstone of diabetes management.

The Benefits of Exercise for Reversal of Type 2 Diabetes

Exercise plays a crucial role in managing and potentially reversing type 2 diabetes. Integrating regular physical activity into your daily routine offers multiple health benefits that directly influence your body's ability to control blood glucose levels and improve overall health. Here are the key benefits of exercise for individuals looking to reverse type 2 diabetes:

Enhances Insulin Sensitivity: Regular physical activity helps your body's cells better respond to insulin. By improving insulin sensitivity, exercise helps decrease the amount of insulin needed to manage blood glucose levels effectively, facilitating easier blood sugar management.

Regulates Blood Glucose Levels: Exercise helps lower blood sugar by encouraging the muscles to use glucose for energy and muscle contraction. This reduction in circulating blood glucose is immediate during and after exercise, and with consistent activity, it can have a long-lasting effect.

Aids in Weight Control: Maintaining a healthy weight is critical for managing diabetes. Exercise burns calories and increases muscle mass, which is essential for weight management. Reducing body fat, particularly around the abdomen, decreases the body's resistance to insulin, making it easier to control diabetes.

Improves Heart Health: Diabetes significantly increases the risk of developing heart disease. Regular exercise strengthens the heart and improves blood circulation, reducing the risk of heart disease and stroke. Activities like aerobic exercises lower blood pressure and improve cholesterol levels.

Reduces Stress: Exercise is an effective stress reliever. It releases endorphins, often referred to as feel-good hormones, which can help alleviate stress, anxiety, and depression—common issues in individuals dealing with chronic conditions like diabetes.

Promotes Overall Well-being: Regular physical activity increases energy levels and overall physical fitness, making daily activities easier and enhancing quality of life. Additionally, exercise contributes to better sleep patterns, which can help regulate hormones and manage diabetes more effectively.

Prevents Diabetes-Related Complications: Exercise can help prevent or delay diabetes-related complications such as neuropathy, retinopathy, and kidney disease by improving blood circulation and reducing cholesterol and blood pressure levels.

Incorporating regular exercise into your lifestyle helps directly manage blood glucose levels and addresses several risk factors associated with long-term complications of diabetes. Whether it's improving heart health, enhancing insulin sensitivity, or controlling weight, the benefits of exercise are extensive and vital for those aiming to reverse type 2 diabetes.

Types of Exercise for Type 2 Diabetes

For individuals managing type 2 diabetes, engaging in various exercises is beneficial for optimizing health and reversing symptoms. Each type of exercise serves different purposes and benefits, providing a comprehensive approach to diabetes management. Here's a straightforward guide to the exercises most beneficial for those with type 2 diabetes.

Aerobic Exercise: Cardiovascular or aerobic exercise is crucial for improving heart health and reducing blood sugar. Walking, cycling, swimming, and jogging help increase heart rate and blood circulation. These exercises use large muscle groups and can be sustained, making them particularly effective for glucose control. Aim for at least 150 minutes of moderate-intensity aerobic activity per week.

Resistance Training: Building and maintaining muscle mass is essential for glucose metabolism. Resistance training such as weightlifting, resistance bands, or bodyweight exercises (like push-ups and squats) helps build muscle, improving insulin sensitivity and muscle glucose uptake. Incorporate resistance training at least two to three times per week.

Flexibility Exercises: Exercises that enhance flexibility, such as yoga and stretching, contribute to better muscle and joint function, which can be affected by high blood sugar levels. Flexibility exercises also aid in reducing stress and improving circulation, further supporting diabetes management.

Balance Training: Balance exercises help prevent falls, essential for individuals with neuropathy (nerve damage) in their feet. Practices like tai chi or simple balance drills (such as standing on one foot) improve stability and coordination.

High-Intensity Interval Training (HIIT): For those who can, HIIT involves short bursts of intense activity followed by a recovery period.

This exercise can significantly improve insulin sensitivity and burn more calories quickly, making it an efficient way to manage diabetes.

Each type of exercise offers unique benefits and can be tailored to individual fitness levels and preferences. Combining different forms of physical activity can help address various aspects of diabetes management more effectively than relying on one type of exercise alone. Always consult with a healthcare provider before starting a new exercise regimen, especially if you have any diabetes-related complications or other health issues.

Starting an Exercise Plan

Beginning an exercise plan can be a daunting task, especially for those with type 2 diabetes who may have specific health considerations. However, with careful planning and a systematic approach, you can effectively incorporate regular physical activity into your diabetes management strategy. Here are essential steps to start an exercise plan that fits your health needs and lifestyle:

Consult with Healthcare Providers: Before starting any new exercise program, consult your doctor or a healthcare professional, particularly if you have any complications associated with diabetes, such as heart problems or neuropathy. They can provide guidelines and restrictions based on your current health condition.

Set Realistic Goals: Define achievable goals based on your fitness level and overall health objectives. Whether walking for 30 minutes a day, swimming twice a week, or simply incorporating more movement into your daily routine, these activities set realistic goals to help keep you motivated and avoid discouragement.

Start Slowly: Begin with low to moderate-intensity activities and gradually increase the intensity and duration as your fitness improves. This gradual progression helps minimize the risk of injury and hypoglycemia, a common concern for those taking insulin or certain oral diabetes medications.

Choose Activities You Enjoy: Exercise doesn't have to be tedious or strenuous. Select activities you enjoy doing, as you are more likely to stick with an exercise plan if it's enjoyable. Consider cycling, dancing, gardening, or even playing a sport.

Create a Balanced Routine: Incorporate a mix of aerobic, resistance, flexibility, and balance exercises to optimize your health benefits. A varied routine addresses different aspects of fitness and keeps the regimen interesting.

Plan for Regularity: Schedule specific times for exercise in your weekly routine to establish consistency, which is crucial for managing diabetes. Consistency in physical activity can help regulate blood sugar levels more effectively.

Monitor Blood Sugar Levels: Check your blood sugar levels before and after exercise to learn how different activities affect your glucose levels. This monitoring is crucial to prevent blood sugar from dropping too low during or after exercise, especially if you are on medications that increase insulin production.

Stay Hydrated and Be Prepared: Always have water on hand to stay hydrated and carry a small carbohydrate-rich snack in case your blood sugar levels drop too low during exercise. Also, wear appropriate footwear and clothing to ensure comfort and prevent injuries.

Be Patient and Flexible: Physical fitness improves gradually, and fluctuations in performance are normal. Be patient with your progress and flexible enough to adjust your exercise plan as needed based on your health status and personal commitments.

Starting an exercise plan for diabetes management is about a lifelong commitment to improving your health. By taking the right precautions, setting achievable goals, and gradually increasing your activity level, you can enjoy the myriad benefits of physical activity in managing and potentially reversing type 2 diabetes.

Pointers to Stay Motivated to Exercise Regularly

Set Clear, Achievable Goals: Define specific, realistic goals you can track over time. These could be a certain number of daily steps, a distance to run without stopping, or a weight to lift. Setting and achieving goals provides a sense of accomplishment and progress.

Track Your Progress: Use a fitness app, journal, or tracker to keep a detailed log of your activities. Monitoring your achievements can significantly increase your motivation by visually documenting your progress.

Vary Your Routine: Mix different activities into your routine to avoid monotony. Alternating between swimming, cycling, group fitness classes, or dance can keep your regimen exciting and cover all aspects of fitness—strength, endurance, flexibility, and balance.

Find an Exercise Partner: Working out with a friend or in a group can make exercising more enjoyable and motivating. It adds a layer of accountability and support, which can be crucial in maintaining a regular schedule.

Reward Yourself: Set up a system to reward yourself for meeting specific targets. Rewards could be anything from new workout gear to a new book, a day out, or a special meal. Rewarding yourself can keep your spirits high and motivate you toward your next milestone.

Stay Positive: Keep a positive outlook on your exercise routine by focusing on the benefits, such as better health, more energy, improved sleep, and a higher sense of well-being. Positive reinforcement is a powerful motivator.

Incorporate It Into Your Daily Schedule: Schedule your workouts like any other important activity. By making them a fixed part of your daily routine, you're more likely to stick to them and less likely to find excuses.

Join a Community: Whether it's an online community or a local exercise group, connecting with others who share similar goals can provide additional motivation. Sharing tips, challenges, and successes with a community can reinforce your commitment to exercising.

Embrace Technology: Utilize apps and online resources to find new workout ideas, track your progress, and engage with fitness communities. Many apps also offer virtual rewards, challenges, and reminders to keep you engaged.

Listen to Your Body: Always be attentive to your feelings during and after workouts. Adjust your exercise intensity and duration to match your current fitness level. Rest when needed to prevent burnout and injuries.

Understand Setbacks Are Part of the Process: Missed workouts or backslides in progress are normal. Every day is a new opportunity to continue pursuing your fitness and health goals.

By applying these motivational strategies, you can sustain your enthusiasm for regular exercise, which is instrumental in managing and potentially reversing type 2 diabetes.

5

Chapter 4

Chapter 4: Medication and Supplements Intervention for Reversing Diabetes

Effective management of type 2 diabetes often requires the use of specific medications and supplements. This chapter explores the options available, how they work within the body, and their potential benefits and side effects. It also covers the role of dietary supplements in diabetes care, providing a comprehensive guide to pharmacological and supplemental interventions.

Overview of Medications Used for Type 2 Diabetes

Metformin: Often the first line of treatment, metformin helps reduce glucose production in the liver and improves the body's sensitivity to insulin.

Sulfonylureas: These stimulate the pancreas to produce more insulin. Examples include glipizide, glyburide, and glimepiride.

Thiazolidinediones: Like metformin, these help improve insulin sensitivity but can have more severe side effects, such as an increased risk of heart problems.

DPP-4 Inhibitors: Drugs like sitagliptin and saxagliptin work by affecting the incretin hormones, which help raise insulin production after meals and decrease the amount of glucose produced by the liver.

GLP-1 Receptor Agonists: This class of drugs improves insulin secretion, slows glucose absorption, and can promote weight loss. Examples include exenatide and liraglutide.

SGLT2 Inhibitors: These help the kidneys lower glucose levels in the blood. Examples include canagliflozin and dapagliflozin.

Insulin Therapy: Insulin therapy is sometimes necessary when other medications are insufficient to control glucose levels. Different formulations can be tailored to manage blood sugar fluctuations throughout the day.

How Medications Operate in the Body

Each class of diabetes medication works through different mechanisms:

- **Insulin Sensitizers** like metformin and thiazolidinediones enhance the body's response to insulin.
- **Insulin Secretagogues** such as sulfonylureas and meglitinides stimulate the pancreas to produce more insulin.
- **Alpha-Glucosidase Inhibitors** slow carbohydrate absorption in the intestines.
- **Peptide Enhancers** like GLP-1 receptor agonists and DPP-4 inhibitors modulate the effect of gut hormones on insulin secretion.
- **SGLT2 Inhibitors** facilitate sugar excretion through the urine.

Understanding these mechanisms helps tailor treatment plans to individual needs, maximizing therapeutic efficacy while minimizing side effects.

The Benefits and Side Effects of Medications

While these medications are effective in managing blood glucose levels, they can also come with side effects:

- **Metformin** may cause gastrointestinal upset but tends to subside over time.
- **Sulfonylureas** can lead to weight gain and an increased risk of hypoglycemia.
- **Thiazolidinediones** are linked to weight gain and more serious issues like heart failure.
- **DPP-4 Inhibitors** are generally well-tolerated but might cause joint pain and skin reactions.
- **GLP-1 Receptor Agonists** can result in gastrointestinal symptoms and are not recommended for people with a history of pancreatitis.
- **SGLT2 Inhibitors** carry risks of urinary tract infections and a rare condition called ketoacidosis.

Balancing these benefits and side effects is a crucial aspect of diabetes management.

Overview of Supplements Used for Type 2 Diabetes

Supplements can also play a role in managing type 2 diabetes:

- **Alpha-lipoic Acid:** Known for its antioxidant properties, it can improve insulin sensitivity and lower blood sugar levels.
- **Magnesium:** Low magnesium levels are typical in people with diabetes; supplements can help improve glucose control.
- **Chromium:** Supplements may enhance insulin sensitivity and glucose metabolism.
- **Omega-3 Fatty Acids:** Helpful in reducing inflammation and improving heart health in people with diabetes.

While supplements can support diabetes treatment, they should not replace medications but rather be used alongside them under the guidance of a healthcare provider.

This chapter provides a foundational understanding of the medications and supplements integral to managing and potentially reversing type 2 diabetes. Understanding the available treatments and how they work allows patients and healthcare providers to make informed decisions that optimize health outcomes.

Overview of Medications Used for Type 2 Diabetes

Effective management of type 2 diabetes often involves the use of various medications, each designed to target different aspects of the disease process. Understanding these medications is crucial for optimizing treatment strategies and improving glucose control. Here's an overview of the primary categories of diabetes medications used to treat type 2 diabetes:

Metformin: One of the most commonly prescribed medications for type 2 diabetes, metformin helps lower glucose production in the liver and improves insulin sensitivity. It's often the first medication prescribed and is known for its efficacy and safety profile.

Sulfonylureas: This class of drugs works by stimulating the beta cells in the pancreas to release more insulin. Examples include glipizide, glyburide, and glimepiride. While effective, they can increase the risk of hypoglycemia and weight gain.

Meglitinides: Like sulfonylureas, meglitinides stimulate insulin secretion from the pancreas but act faster and shorter. They are taken before meals to control postprandial blood sugar spikes.

Thiazolidinediones (TZDs): These drugs increase insulin sensitivity and reduce glucose production in the liver. Examples include piogli-tazone and rosiglitazone. However, they can have side effects such as weight gain and increased risk of heart failure.

DPP-4 Inhibitors: These medications block the enzyme dipeptidyl peptidase-4, which prolongs incretin hormone activity, increases insulin release, and decreases glucagon levels in the blood. Examples include sitagliptin, saxagliptin, and linagliptin.

GLP-1 Receptor Agonists: These injectable medications mimic the incretin hormones that the body usually produces after a meal, which enhances insulin secretion, suppresses glucagon release, and slows gastric emptying. Examples include exenatide, liraglutide, and dulaglutide.

SGLT2 Inhibitors: Sodium-glucose cotransporter 2 inhibitors work by preventing the kidneys from reabsorbing glucose back into the blood. This leads to reduced blood sugar levels and possible weight loss. Examples include canagliflozin, dapagliflozin, and empagliflozin.

Insulin Therapy: While many people with type 2 diabetes may not need insulin initially, some may require it to manage their blood sugar effectively, especially as the disease progresses—insulin therapy tailors with different types of insulin to manage blood sugar fluctuations throughout the day.

These medications can be used alone or in combination, depending on individual needs and specific diabetes management goals. Patients should work closely with their healthcare providers to determine the best medication plan based on their unique health profile, lifestyle, and glucose control needs.

How Medications Operate in the Body

Understanding how diabetes medications operate within the body is crucial for effectively managing type 2 diabetes. Each class of drugs targets different pathways to help control blood sugar levels, improve insulin sensitivity, or mimic hormonal interactions. Here's a concise breakdown of how these medications work:

Metformin: Metformin primarily reduces the amount of glucose released by the liver. It also enhances the sensitivity of muscle cells to insulin, allowing them to remove more glucose from the blood, thus improving overall blood sugar control.

Sulfonylureas and Meglitinides: Both medications stimulate the beta cells of the pancreas to produce more insulin. Sulfonylureas have a more prolonged action duration than meglitinides, which act quickly and for a shorter period. This makes them helpful in managing blood sugar levels around meal times.

Thiazolidinediones (TZDs): TZDs improve insulin sensitivity in muscle and fat cells, making them more effective at absorbing glucose. They also mildly suppress glucose production in the liver. However, their use is sometimes limited due to side effects related to weight gain and cardiovascular risks.

DPP-4 Inhibitors: These medications help prolong the action of incretin hormones released after eating and signal the pancreas to produce more insulin and less glucagon (a hormone that raises blood glucose levels). DPP-4 inhibitors lead to an increase in insulin secretion and a decrease in glucagon secretion, mainly when glucose levels are high.

GLP-1 Receptor Agonists: This class of injectables enhances the incretin system in a way similar to DPP-4 inhibitors but more directly by mimicking the effects of GLP-1, a natural hormone. They boost insulin release, suppress glucagon production, and slow digestion, which helps prevent large spikes in blood sugar after meals.

SGLT2 Inhibitors: These medications block glucose reabsorption in the kidneys, promoting the excretion of excess glucose through the urine. This helps lower blood glucose levels and can reduce weight loss and blood pressure.

Insulin Therapy: Insulin therapy is used when the body no longer produces enough insulin or when other medications are insufficient to control glucose levels. Insulin therapy directly supplements the body's insulin, helping transport glucose into cells for energy and lowering blood sugar levels.

Each medication interacts with the body's natural processes in specific ways to lower blood sugar levels, improve metabolic health, and mitigate the effects of diabetes. The choice of medication, or combination, depends on individual factors such as the patient's specific health conditions, the degree of blood sugar control needed, and how the body responds to treatment. Understanding these mechanisms helps tailor treatment to achieve optimal diabetes management.

The Benefits and Side Effects of Medications

Diabetes medications are vital for managing type 2 diabetes but come with both benefits and potential side effects. Understanding these can help in making informed treatment decisions.

Benefits of Diabetes Medications

Enhanced Glycemic Control: These medications effectively lower blood glucose levels, helping to prevent diabetes-related complications.

Reduced Risk of Complications: Proper blood sugar management reduces the risks associated with diabetes, such as heart disease, neuropathy, and kidney damage.

Weight Management: Some medications, like GLP-1 receptor agonists and SGLT2 inhibitors, can aid in weight loss, benefiting overall diabetes management.

Increased Insulin Production: Drugs such as sulfonylureas boost insulin output from the pancreas, improving blood sugar management.

Improved Insulin Sensitivity: Medications like metformin enhance the body's responsiveness to insulin, aiding in more effective blood sugar regulation.

Side Effects of Diabetes Medications

Hypoglycemia: Medications that increase insulin can lead to dangerously low blood sugar levels.

Weight Gain: Some drugs, including insulin and oral medications, may cause weight gain, complicating diabetes management.

Gastrointestinal Discomfort: Common with metformin, side effects include nausea and diarrhea, especially when starting treatment.

Cardiovascular Risks: Certain medications may increase the risk of heart disease or heart failure.

Infections: SGLT2 inhibitors increase the risk for genital and urinary tract infections due to increased sugar in the urine.

Bone Density Issues: Long-term use of some diabetes drugs can lead to decreased bone density and increased fracture risk.

Pancreatitis: GLP-1 receptor agonists are associated with a rare risk of pancreatitis.

While diabetes medications effectively control the condition, monitoring for side effects is crucial for safety. Continuous collaboration with healthcare providers is necessary to adjust treatment plans to optimize benefits and minimize risks.

Overview of Supplements Used for Type 2 Diabetes

While medications are the cornerstone of type 2 diabetes management, certain dietary supplements can also play a supportive role in controlling the condition. Here's a concise overview of the common supplements that may benefit individuals with type 2 diabetes, focusing on how they work and their potential benefits.

Alpha-Lipoic Acid (ALA): ALA is a powerful antioxidant that can help improve insulin sensitivity and reduce symptoms of diabetic neuropathy, such as pain, burning, and numbness in the legs and arms. It works by combating oxidative stress, a critical factor in the deterioration of diabetes complications.

Chromium: This essential trace element enhances insulin's action and is involved in carbohydrate, fat, and protein metabolism. Supplementing with chromium may improve glucose tolerance and reduce blood sugar levels.

Magnesium: Magnesium plays a crucial role in glucose control and insulin metabolism. Diabetic individuals often have lower magnesium levels, and supplementation can help improve glucose levels and insulin sensitivity.

Omega-3 Fatty Acids: In fish oil and flaxseeds, omega-3s can help lower triglyceride levels and elevate HDL (good) cholesterol levels, essential for heart health in people with diabetes. They also help reduce inflammation and improve cellular function.

Vitamin D: Adequate vitamin D levels are essential for calcium metabolism and general health. Some studies suggest that vitamin D may help improve insulin sensitivity and beta-cell function.

Bitter Melon: Often used in traditional medicine, bitter melon helps lower blood glucose levels. Some components in bitter melon may act similarly to insulin, allowing glucose to move into cells for energy.

Cinnamon: Some studies suggest that cinnamon may reduce fasting blood glucose levels and improve insulin sensitivity by mimicking the effects of insulin and increasing glucose transport into cells.

Fenugreek: Rich in soluble fiber, which helps lower blood sugar by slowing down carbohydrate digestion and absorption. Regular use of fenugreek might be effective in controlling diabetes.

While these supplements can offer potential benefits, they are not a substitute for diabetes medication and should not be used as the primary treatment. It's crucial for anyone considering these supplements to consult with their healthcare provider to ensure they are appropriate and safe, mainly because some supplements can interact with medications and affect blood sugar levels unpredictably. Also, efficacy varies from person to person based on individual health conditions and the nature of their diabetes management plan.

6

Chapter 5

Chapter 5: **Monitoring Your Diabetes and Self-Care for Reversing Diabetes**

Effective management and potential reversal of type 2 diabetes hinge significantly on diligent self-monitoring and comprehensive self-care. This chapter delves into the crucial practices of monitoring blood glucose levels and adopting various self-care strategies to manage and potentially reverse diabetes.

The Importance of Monitoring Blood Glucose Levels

Regular monitoring of blood glucose levels is essential for managing type 2 diabetes. It helps in:

- **Identifying Patterns and Trends:** Tracking glucose levels over time can reveal the effects of dietary choices, physical activity, and medications on blood sugar.
- **Adjusting Treatment Plans:** Frequent monitoring allows for timely adjustments in medication, diet, and exercise, optimizing diabetes management.
- **Preventing Complications:** Maintaining blood sugar levels within target ranges can reduce the risk of long-term complications such

as neuropathy, retinopathy, and kidney disease.

- **Empowering Self-Management:** Regular monitoring enhances your understanding of diabetes and your body's response to different management strategies, promoting a proactive approach to care.

Overview of Self-Care Techniques for Type 2 Diabetes

Self-care for diabetes involves several routine practices that not only help manage the disease but also improve overall health:

- **Dietary Management:** Consistent with the guidance in earlier chapters, maintaining a balanced diet is crucial.
- **Regular Exercise:** As detailed previously, regular physical activity helps improve insulin sensitivity and cardiovascular health.
- **Stress Management:** Chronic stress can negatively affect blood sugar levels and overall health. Techniques such as mindfulness, meditation, and adequate sleep are beneficial.
- **Regular Check-Ups:** Frequent visits to healthcare providers for comprehensive check-ups help catch and mitigate complications early.

Management of a Sick Day

Illness can cause significant fluctuations in blood sugar levels, making diabetes challenging to control. During sick days, it's essential to:

- **Monitor Blood Glucose More Frequently:** Illness, especially fever, can increase blood glucose levels. More frequent testing can help manage unexpected shifts.
- **Stay Hydrated:** Illness often leads to fluid loss, and dehydration can impact blood sugar levels and treatment efficacy.
- **Adjust Medication If Needed:** Consult a healthcare provider about adjusting insulin dosage or other medications during illness.

- **Have a Sick Day Plan:** Prepare a plan in consultation with your healthcare provider, including when to take medication, what to eat, how often to check your glucose, and when to call a doctor.

Traveling with Diabetes

Traveling requires special preparations to manage diabetes effectively:

- **Pack Adequate Supplies:** Ensure you have enough medication, testing supplies, and snacks for the entire trip, plus extra in case of travel delays.
- **Maintain Meal and Medication Schedules:** Stick to your regular meal and medication schedules as much as possible.
- **Carry Medical Identification:** Always have a form of medical identification that mentions your diabetes in case of an emergency.
- **Know How to Store Medication:** Certain medications, particularly insulin, must be stored properly to maintain effectiveness. Research how to store your medication while traveling.

This chapter highlights the critical roles of monitoring and self-care in managing type 2 diabetes. By understanding and implementing these strategies, individuals with diabetes can take significant steps toward reversing their condition and enhancing their quality of life.

The Importance of Monitoring Blood Glucose Levels

Regular monitoring of blood glucose levels is a cornerstone of effective diabetes management and can be pivotal in reversing type 2 diabetes. This practice provides critical insights into how different factors such as diet, physical activity, medications, and stress affect your blood sugar levels. Here are the key reasons why consistent monitoring is essential:

Enables Immediate Feedback: Monitoring your glucose levels offers immediate feedback on your health status. This information allows you to understand how your lifestyle choices and medications influence your blood sugar levels, helping you make immediate corrections if needed.

Helps Optimize Treatment Plans: Regular glucose checks help fine-tune your diabetes management plan. They provide your healthcare team with detailed data to make informed decisions about medication, diet, and exercise adjustments. This customization is crucial for effectively managing diabetes and preventing complications.

Aids in Preventing Complications: Keeping blood glucose levels within a target range can significantly reduce the risk of developing long-term diabetes complications such as nerve damage, kidney disease, and cardiovascular problems. Regular monitoring ensures your glucose levels are stable and within safe limits.

Increases Self-awareness and Empowerment: By regularly checking your blood sugar levels, you become more attuned to your body's responses to different foods, activities, and stressors. This increased awareness empowers you to take control of your health and make lifestyle choices that positively impact your diabetes management.

Supports Lifestyle Adjustments: Monitoring can help you see the benefits of healthy lifestyle changes reflected in your blood sugar levels. This positive reinforcement can motivate adherence to beneficial practices such as healthy eating and regular physical activity.

Detects Hypoglycemia and Hyperglycemia: Frequent monitoring is crucial to detect and respond to hypoglycemia (low blood sugar) and hyperglycemia (high blood sugar), which can be dangerous if not addressed promptly. Understanding these trends allows for timely interventions, which can prevent emergencies.

In summary, regular monitoring of blood glucose levels is invaluable in managing type 2 diabetes. It helps fine-tune treatment and prevent complications and empowers individuals with diabetes to take active control of their health, leading to improved outcomes and potentially reversing the course of the disease.

Overview of Self-Care Techniques for Type 2 Diabetes

Effective self-care is crucial for individuals with type 2 diabetes. It involves a comprehensive approach that includes lifestyle management, daily monitoring, and preventive practices to manage symptoms and enhance overall health. Here are the essential self-care techniques that every person with type 2 diabetes should consider incorporating into their daily routine:

Dietary Management: Adhering to a balanced diet rich in nutrients, low in unhealthy fats and sugars, and moderate in calories is essential. Focus on incorporating whole grains, lean proteins, healthy fats, and plenty of fruits and vegetables to help regulate blood sugar levels.

Physical Activity: Regular exercise is crucial as it helps to lower blood sugar levels, reduce body fat, and improve heart health. Aim for at least 150 minutes of moderate aerobic activity each week, supplemented by strength training exercises two to three times weekly.

Regular Blood Sugar Monitoring: Consistently checking your blood glucose levels allows you to adjust your diet, exercise, and medications based on real-time data. This frequent monitoring helps maintain glucose levels within the target range your healthcare provider prescribes.

Proper Medication Adherence: Take all medications as prescribed by your healthcare provider. Understanding how your medications work and their possible side effects can help you manage your condition more effectively.

Stress Management: Stress can significantly impact blood glucose levels. Deep breathing, yoga, meditation, and mindfulness can effectively manage stress and stabilize blood sugar levels.

Adequate Sleep: Good sleep hygiene is essential, as poor sleep can affect blood sugar levels and insulin sensitivity. Aim for 7-9 hours of quality sleep per night and maintain a regular sleep schedule.

Foot Care: Daily foot inspections are necessary to avoid complications such as infections, ulcers, and even amputations. Check for cuts, blisters, redness, and swelling.

Regular Health Check-ups: Regular visits to your healthcare provider for comprehensive check-ups can help catch and manage complications early. These should include primary care visits, regular eye exams, dental check-ups, and screenings for neuropathy.

Avoiding Smoking and Limiting Alcohol: Smoking and excessive alcohol consumption can exacerbate diabetes complications. If you smoke, seek help to quit, and if you drink alcohol, do so in moderation, following the guidelines provided by your healthcare provider.

Education and Support: Stay informed about new research and treatment options for type 2 diabetes. Joining support groups and diabetes education programs can also provide motivation and improve your ability to manage the disease.

By implementing these self-care techniques, individuals with type 2 diabetes can significantly improve their quality of life and overall health outcomes. These practices help manage the disease daily and play a crucial role in preventing the long-term complications associated with diabetes.

Management of a Sick Day for Type 2 Diabetes

Illness can significantly impact blood glucose levels, making diabetes management more challenging. Proper planning and effective strategies are essential to handle sick days without exacerbating your condition. Here's how to manage diabetes effectively when you're not feeling well:

Monitor Blood Glucose More Frequently: Illness, particularly fever, stress, or infection, can lead to fluctuations in blood sugar levels. It's crucial to monitor these levels more frequently during sick days, as you may need to adjust your medication or insulin dosage accordingly.

Stay Hydrated: Dehydration is a risk with increased blood glucose levels, and it's more likely if you're experiencing fever, vomiting, or diarrhea. Drink plenty of fluids to stay hydrated. Opt for water and avoid sugary drinks, which can spike blood sugar levels. If your blood sugar levels are high, consider fluids low in carbohydrates and calories.

Continue Medications: Don't stop taking your diabetes medication unless your healthcare provider advises you to. If you're unable to eat your normal diet, contact your healthcare provider for specific instructions on medication adjustments. This is especially important for insulin users, as dosages might need to be adjusted.

Easy-to-Digest Foods: If your regular meal plan is not feasible, try to consume easy-to-digest foods that help maintain carbohydrate intake. Suitable options include unsweetened applesauce, plain crackers, broth, and boiled potatoes. If you cannot eat solid food, consider liquid carbohydrate-containing foods like clear soups or natural fruit juices to maintain energy levels.

Check for Ketones: If your blood sugar is consistently high (typically over 240 mg/dL), check your urine for ketones with an over-the-counter test kit. The presence of ketones indicates that your body is using fat for energy instead of glucose, a condition that can lead to diabetic ketoacidosis, a potentially life-threatening complication.

Rest: Give your body enough rest to recover. Physical stress from illness can increase blood sugar levels, so managing your health with adequate rest is essential.

Develop a Sick Day Plan: Before you get sick, developing a sick day plan in consultation with your healthcare provider is wise. This plan should include which medications to continue, how often to check your blood sugar and ketones, when to adjust your medication doses, and when to call your healthcare provider.

Communicate With Your Healthcare Provider: Contact your healthcare provider if you notice significant changes in your symptoms or cannot keep fluids or foods down. Professional guidance is crucial in preventing complications.

By following these guidelines, you can manage your diabetes more effectively during sick days and prevent minor illnesses from becoming severe complications.

Traveling with Diabetes

Traveling with type 2 diabetes requires careful planning to manage your condition effectively while away from home. Here are focused strategies to ensure that diabetes management remains consistent, even on the move:

Plan Ahead: Before you travel, consult with your healthcare provider to discuss your travel plans and any necessary adjustments to your medication schedule, especially if you'll be crossing time zones, which could affect medication timing.

Carry a Diabetes Travel Letter: Obtain a letter from your healthcare provider detailing your diabetes medications, supplies, and allergies. This document can be helpful during security checks and in case of emergency abroad.

Pack Extra Supplies: Always pack more medication and testing supplies than you need, accounting for potential delays or loss. Include extra batteries for your glucose meter, insulin pens, syringes, and other necessities.

Keep Medications with You: Always carry your medications, including insulin, in your carry-on luggage to avoid extreme temperatures in checked baggage and ensure access if your luggage is lost. Medications should be in their original prescription bottles with labels.

Store Insulin Properly: If you use insulin, ensure it is stored correctly. Most manufacturers recommend storing it at room temperature once it is used. However, for long-term storage, insulin should be refrigerated. Consider carrying an insulated bag with cooling packs if traveling to a hot climate.

Maintain Your Meal Schedule: To manage your blood sugar, stick to your usual meal times as closely as possible. Bring snacks you typically eat in case suitable food options are unavailable.

Stay Hydrated: Carry a water bottle and drink regularly. Dehydration can affect blood sugar levels, and it's easier to become dehydrated while traveling.

Wear Medical Identification: Always wear medical identification that states you have diabetes. Medical identification can be invaluable in the event of a health emergency.

Monitor Blood Sugar Frequently: Changes in activity, meal patterns, and time zones can affect your blood sugar levels. Check your levels more frequently than at home to catch and address any significant fluctuations early.

Be Aware of New Activities: Travel often involves more physical activity than usual, whether sightseeing or walking; anticipate these changes that might affect your blood glucose and plan accordingly.

Know Local Medical Facilities: Before traveling, identify where to access medical care at your destination if needed. Know the generic names of your medications since brand names can vary internationally.

By carefully preparing and maintaining awareness of how travel can impact your diabetes, you can manage your condition effectively while enjoying your travels. This approach ensures that diabetes doesn't have to be a barrier to exploring new places and experiences.

7

Chapter 6

Chapter 6: Tips and Success Stories for Reversal of Type 2 Diabetes

Successfully managing and potentially reversing type 2 diabetes requires dedication, informed strategies, and continuous motivation. This chapter provides practical advice and inspiring success stories to encourage and guide those on their journey to better health.

Strategies and Tips for Staying on Track with the Management of Diabetes

Create a Routine: Establish a daily routine that includes regular meal times, scheduled medication intakes, consistent exercise periods, and blood glucose monitoring. A routine helps reinforce habits that are critical for managing diabetes effectively.

Set Achievable Goals: Break your long-term health objectives into smaller, manageable goals. Achievable milestones, such as a slight reduction in A1C levels, increasing daily steps, or weight loss, can provide a sense of accomplishment and propel you forward.

Utilize Technology: Smartphone apps can help you track food intake, physical activity, and blood glucose levels. Many apps also offer reminders to take medication and stay active.

Educate Yourself: Continuously educate yourself about diabetes management. Understanding the latest research and treatment options can empower you to make informed decisions about your health.

Prepare for Challenges: Anticipate potential challenges such as holiday feasts or travel. Plan how to handle these situations in advance by adjusting your meal plan, medication, or exercise schedule.

Seek Support: Connect with others who are managing diabetes. Support groups, whether online or in-person, can provide invaluable advice, empathy, and motivation from people who understand your challenges.

Regular Medical Check-ups: Keep regular appointments with your healthcare team. These check-ups are crucial for monitoring your health status and making necessary adjustments to your treatment plan.

Motivation and Encouragement for Readers

Success Stories: Sharing the success stories of individuals who have effectively managed or reversed their type 2 diabetes motivates others with diabetes. These stories highlight the strategies that worked, the challenges faced, and how they were overcome, providing inspiration and real-world proof that managing diabetes is achievable.

Celebrate Small Victories: Every step in the right direction is worth celebrating. Whether improving your diet, losing weight, or lowering your blood glucose levels, acknowledging these victories can boost your morale and motivation.

Focus on the Benefits: Consider the benefits of managing diabetes, not just avoiding complications. Improved energy levels, better physical health, enhanced well-being, and a greater sense of control over your life are all powerful motivators.

Stay Positive: Diabetes management is a journey with ups and downs. Maintaining a positive outlook can help you deal with setbacks more effectively and stay committed to your health goals.

Visualize Success: Imagine the life you will lead once you have your diabetes under better control. Visualization is a potent tool for staying motivated and focused on your goals.

This chapter aims to arm readers with practical strategies and motivational insights to help them remain diligent in their diabetes management efforts. Through careful planning, ongoing education, and a supportive community, reversing type 2 diabetes can be attainable, leading to a healthier and more fulfilling life.

Strategies and Tips for Staying on Track with the Management of Diabetes

Successfully managing diabetes requires a consistent and proactive approach. Here are practical strategies and tips designed to help individuals with type 2 diabetes stay on track with their diabetes management:

Establish a Daily Routine: Create a structured daily schedule with specific meal times, exercise, medication, and glucose monitoring. Consistency helps stabilize blood sugar levels and makes management more straightforward and less stressful.

Set Specific Goals: Break your long-term diabetes management goals into smaller, measurable, and achievable objectives. Your goals might include setting targets for daily physical activity, dietary goals for each meal, or glucose level targets to hit each month.

Embrace Technology: Use digital tools and apps to track blood sugar levels, dietary intake, and physical activity. Many apps also provide reminders for taking medication and tips for maintaining a healthy lifestyle.

Stay Educated: Keep up-to-date with the latest diabetes research and treatment options. Understanding your condition dramatically increases your ability to make informed decisions about your health.

Prepare for Challenges: Anticipate situations that could disrupt your routine, such as travel, holidays, or busy periods at work. Adjust your meal planning, medication, or exercise regimen to accommodate these changes.

Build a Support Network: Surround yourself with people who understand and support your journey with diabetes. This could include family, friends, healthcare providers, or support groups. Sharing experiences and solutions can provide emotional support and valuable insights.

Keep Regular Check-ups: Regular appointments with your healthcare team are essential for tracking your progress and making necessary adjustments to your treatment plan. These check-ups often motivate you as you see tangible results from your management efforts.

Monitor Your Progress: Regularly review your progress toward your goals. This can involve tracking your blood glucose levels, noting improvements in your A1C results, or celebrating weight loss achievements. Based on your progress, adjust your goals as needed.

Develop Coping Strategies: Managing diabetes can be stressful. Develop healthy coping strategies, such as practicing meditation, engaging in hobbies, or exercising. Reducing stress is beneficial for blood sugar control.

Stay Flexible: Be prepared to adapt your management plan as your health needs change over time. Flexibility can help you maintain control over your diabetes long-term despite the inevitable changes in life and health.

By implementing these strategies, individuals with type 2 diabetes can enhance their ability to manage the disease effectively. Staying informed, prepared, and connected is critical to successful diabetes management.

Motivation and Encouragement for Readers

Managing type 2 diabetes is a long-term commitment that requires consistent effort and adaptation. Staying motivated and maintaining a positive outlook are essential for successful management. Here are focused strategies to provide motivation and encouragement for individuals managing diabetes:

Celebrate Small Wins: Recognize and celebrate every success along your diabetes management journey, no matter how small. Whether it's sticking to your diet, exercising regularly, or achieving a blood sugar target, acknowledging these victories can boost your morale and motivate you.

Connect with Success Stories: Reading or hearing about others who have successfully managed or reversed their diabetes can be incredibly inspiring. These stories can provide practical insights and demonstrate that your goals are achievable.

Set Realistic Expectations: Understand that progress may be slow and setbacks can occur. Setting realistic expectations can help prevent feelings of discouragement and help you stay committed to your health goals.

Find Your 'Why': Have a clear and personal reason for managing your diabetes effectively—whether it's to enjoy a healthier lifestyle, be active with your family, or achieve a personal health milestone. Reminding yourself of this reason can keep you driven and focused.

Involve Your Loved Ones: Share your goals and plans with friends and family. Their understanding, support, and encouragement can be crucial, especially on difficult days.

Join a Community: Whether online or in-person, communities of others managing diabetes can provide support, advice, and camaraderie. Knowing you are not alone in your journey can be a powerful motivator.

Visualize Your Success: Regularly visualize yourself achieving your goals and living a healthy life. Visualization is a powerful mental exercise that can increase your motivation to pursue and stick to your management plan.

Educate Yourself: Continuous learning about diabetes and its management can empower you. Education enables you to make informed decisions and keep up with new tools or treatments that could improve your quality of life.

Keep a Positive Attitude: Try to maintain a positive attitude about your diabetes management. Positive thinking can positively influence your mental and physical health and make managing diabetes feel less burdensome.

Reward Yourself: Set up a reward system for meeting certain milestones. Rewards can include a new book, a small trip, a new piece of clothing, or anything else that might signify a personal treat.

These motivational strategies can help you maintain enthusiasm and commitment to your diabetes management plan. Remember, each day is a new opportunity to take steps toward a healthier future, and your efforts are the building blocks of a successful strategy.

8

Conclusion

As we conclude this journey through "Reverse Diabetes: Practical Strategies, Diet Plans, and Lifestyle Changes to Beat Diabetes," it's important to reflect on the essential message of empowerment and hope that resonates throughout this book. While type 2 diabetes is a serious and potentially debilitating disease, it offers the possibility of reversal or significant management through informed, proactive steps.

We've explored how a combination of dietary adjustments, regular physical activity, diligent medication management, and vigilant self-care can radically improve your health and potentially reverse the effects of diabetes. These strategies aren't just theoretical; they're practical, attainable, and supported by scientific research and the success stories of individuals who have walked this path before you.

Remember, the journey to reverse diabetes is a personal one. It requires commitment, consistency, and the willingness to make sometimes difficult changes in your lifestyle. But the rewards—improved health, increased vitality, and reduced diabetes-related complications—are profound and life-altering.

As you move forward, remember that small, daily actions can lead to significant results. Regularly monitoring your blood glucose levels, stay-ing active, eating well, and keeping up with your medical appointments are all part of a comprehensive approach to diabetes management.

Finally, I encourage you to share your journey and the insights you've gained from this book with others. If you found value in the strategies and stories shared within these pages, please leave a review on Amazon. Your feedback not only helps us improve but also inspires and guides others who are seeking to manage or reverse their diabetes.

You are on your way towards a healthier future. Remember, each day brings a new opportunity to improve your health and take control of your diabetes. Here's to your health and success on this journey!

9

Resources

OpenAI. (2021). ChatGPT (GPT-3.5) [Software]. OpenAI. https://www.openai.com/